Intermittent Fasting For Women

The Ultimate Beginner's Guide to Fast Weight Loss, Fat Burn, and A Healthy Longer Life.

By Jennifer Louissa

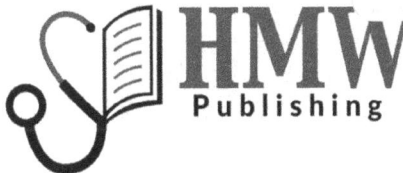

HMW Publishing

For more great books visit:

HMWPublishing.com

Get another book for Free

I want to thank you for purchasing this book and offer you another book (just as long and valuable as this book), "Health & Fitness Mistakes You Don't Know You're Making", completely free.

Visit the link below to signup and receive it:

www.hmwpublishing.com/gift

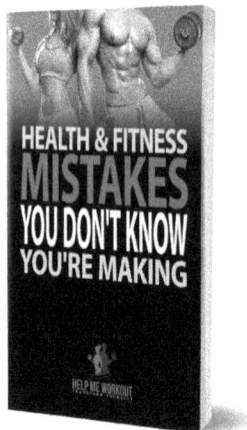

In this book, I will break down the most common health & fitness mistakes, you are probably committing right now, and I will reveal how you can easily get in the best shape of your life!

In addition to this valuable gift, you will also have an opportunity to get our new books for free, enter giveaways, and receive other valuable emails from me. Again, visit the link to sign up: www.hmwpublishing.com/ gift

Table of Contents

Introduction

This book, *Intermittent Fasting for Women: The Ultimate Women's Guide to Intermittent Fasting*, has useful and practical information that will help you get started on intermittent fasting that is specially tuned to your womanly needs.

It is really quite a hassle for women, especially those who are busy juggling work and family to focus on losing weight. This is because most diet routine out there relies on counting the calories that you eat and it's quite a hassle to log and count every single food you eat just so you can be sure that you are not eating beyond your calorie limit.

With this type of dieting, most women end up quitting because they just couldn't commit to too much fuzz. This is where intermittent fasting comes in. With this kind of dieting method, you don't have to worry too much about what you are eating because the method focuses more on "When" you eat and not on "What" you eat. The number of people who have found success in this method is increasing and if you want to be one of those people, then this book will help you. This is the very purpose of this book—to give women, like you, a resource of information on how to start with intermittent fasting.

Men and women have different dieting needs. The intermittent fasting specifics that is tailored for a man may not work as well as it should on women. This is where this book comes in. You will find here useful and practical information that will help you begin the intermittent fasting journey that is tailored to the specifications of women like you.

What is Intermittent Fasting?

There are a lot of dieting fads and health trends that people try out these days. The newest, and perhaps the most unusual yet an effective choice is Intermittent Fasting. So, what makes intermittent fasting stand out from the other diet regimens out there? Well, for starters, intermittent fasting is not a matter of "What" but a matter of "When".

Intermittent fasting is more of an eating pattern than a diet scheme. Weight loss is only among the great side effects. Essentially, with intermittent fasting, you cycle between eating and fasting. There is no specific boundary or limit with what you can eat, rather, it is focused more on when you should eat. There are a lot of methods of intermittent fasting, these methods vary according to how long the fasting cycle is. These cycles split the week, or the day, into eating and fasting hours. For women, it is recommended that the cycle between eating and fasting is not set too steep because the female body is more averse to changes than men. A 14-hour fasting and 10-hour eating cycle is a good start for women while men can start with a bit longer cycle like the 16/8.

What makes this method interesting is that it taps into the very core of human feeding habits. A regular person "fasts" during sleep, meaning there is no feed intake. Intermittent fasting simply extends that length of fasting. There are also people who, due to hectic schedules, skip breakfast or lunch and just nibble on snacks in between. This is already fasting. For example, if you skip your breakfast, eat your first meal of the day at lunch, and dinner as the last sustenance, you are already foregoing 16 hours of eating and restricting your eating into an 8-hour window. This type of meal skipping is part of the 16/8 protocol of intermittent fasting.

You see, humans have been fasting for years. Some may do it for religion or to conserve a limited resource. When sick, humans instinctively fast to prevent further altercations. Fasting is just a natural process that the body is well-acquainted with. There are just some cases where the body needs to adapt first especially if a person is not used to prolonged fasting. But once the body adapts, fasting will become easier.

Who is Intermittent Fasting For?

A lot of women keep on asking, is intermittent fasting effective? And if so, is it for me? Can I do intermittent fasting without harmful repercussions?

Who CAN DO intermittent fasting?

Well, generally, anyone can do intermittent fasting, given that they are healthy. If you are not suffering on any illness that requires you to maintain or sustain a lot of nutrients or is not allowed to suffer any fluctuations in weight, then intermittent fasting may be a thing for you.

However, extra caution and supervision may be needed for those who have diabetes mellitus (Type 1 and 2), taking prescription medication, or have high uric acid or gout. If you are suffering or currently doing any of those, then it is recommended that you consult with your doctor first on whether you can engage in intermittent fasting.

Who CANNOT DO intermittent fasting?

Even when intermittent fasting is for anyone who can do it, there are still some limitations as well. You can't engage in intermittent fasting if:

You are underweight.

Being underweight is one reason why you should not do fasting. A BMI of less than 18.5 is generally considered underweight for both men and women. However, men have a lower fat percentage than women so 14-17% fat ratio is still considered normal while lesser than that is underweight. Women need about 21-33% of fat to fit the normal weight ratio. With this slightly higher percentage requirement than men, if you fall under the underweight category, losing even more weight will only make things worse for you. Instead, focus more on increasing your weight to normal rather than fasting to lose even more.

You are pregnant.

If you are pregnant, you cannot afford to lose those nutrients because you will need them to sustain yourself and your child. If you really plan to engage in intermittent fasting, make sure to do so after you have given birth and with approval from your doctor.

You are breastfeeding.

When you are breastfeeding or still nursing your child, you cannot engage in intermittent fasting. Your child needs as many nutrients and vitamins that will help him/her grow and develop, and he/she gets the nutrients from breastfeeding. If you are doing intermittent fasting while nursing your baby, it may affect the quality and amount of nutrients available for him/her.

You are under 18.

No matter how much you want to lose weight while you are a teenager, intermittent fasting is not recommended for you. You need as much nutrition to grow and intermittent fasting cuts that. It may hamper your growth. Wait a few more years, or at least until you are 18, and consult adults if you really want to do this.

Chapter 1: Understanding Intermittent Fasting

Just like all dieting fads, intermittent fasting is not immune to doubts and questions from health experts and customers alike. Some question on whether or not the claims that surround intermittent fasting actually have a scientific basis or they are just hearsay. These questions ensue because people have begun to gather opposing thoughts on the method. Even when the method first arose with origins backed by legitimate science, the details become exaggerated by the time it hits mainstream popularity. This is what is happening with intermittent fasting now. Even when the idea is backed with scientific evidence, due to the increasing number of unwarranted claims, the concept has been a receiving both good and bad retorts. Well, this book will help clear out the misconceptions.

The Science Behind Intermittent Fasting

Intermittent fasting is anchored on the idea that fasting helps promote better health. This idea is backed by numerous studies and evidence that have been conducted for years. According to these studies, fasting has been known to improve the well-being of a person such as reducing the impact of stress, improving memory, improving cardiovascular health, weight loss and more.

Mark Mattson, a senior investigator of the US National Institute on Aging under the National Institute of Health, explored the benefits of intermittent fasting and gathered significant evidence to the claim. The investigations conducted targeted the effect of intermittent fasting on neurons and brain health, weight loss, and markers of stress. Results of these studies show significant improvement in the cases of the participants. These findings were also supported by more studies with the same focus and more [1, 2, 3].

More and more studies are being conducted to further cement the benefits of intermittent fasting to human health. However, precautions are still being taken to promote the legitimate strategies that fall under the system to ensure that those who plan to follow the trend end up following something authentic and not just a fad made-up by those who want to get into the bandwagon of fame.[1]

[1] Collier, R. (2013). Intermittent fasting: the science of going without.

[2] Barnosky, A. R., Hoddy, K. K., Unterman, T. G., & Varady, K. A. (2014). Intermittent fasting vs daily calorie restriction for type 2 diabetes prevention: a review of human findings. *Translational Research*, *164*(4), 302-311.

[3] Rudman, D., Feller, A. G., Nagraj, H. S., Gergans, G. A., Lalitha, P. Y., Goldberg, A. F., ... & Mattson, D. E. (1990). Effects of human growth hormone in men over 60 years old. *New England Journal of Medicine*, *323*(1), 1-6.

Understanding the Risks of Intermittent Fasting

It is important to note that as much as how beneficial intermittent fasting has become, there are still risks that women, like you, need to consider. These risks may or may not occur to you as you proceed with fasting, but it is never a bad thing to consider them nonetheless. The knowledge of these risks will help you practice caution as you fast intermittently.

You elevate your cortisol levels.

When you do intermittent fasting, you are urging your body to force it to use fat as the main source of energy. This induces stress to your body and as the process becomes more stressful, the level of the stress hormone, cortisol, also increases. If this elevation in cortisol persists, it may lead to negative effects such as the breakdown of muscles and increased fat.

You can get unhealthily obsessed with food.

At first, when you enter intermittent fasting, your main goal is to probably lose weight and improve your general health. However, as you progress with your fasting, you may eventually develop an unhealthy obsession with food. Not eating food per se but thinking about it. As you see your friends take their scrumptious lunches or breakfast, your hunger will end up driving you into planning which meals to take that will keep you full and not forgo fasting, or even think about skipping. Your mind becomes filled with nothing but food due to hunger that you won't notice that you've already forgotten about that file that your boss needs or that appointment you need to set-up. Everything else takes the backseat as food hoards that shotgun.

You may end up relying on coffee too much.

Coffee is the go-to drink for those who are too busy to get proper food. Coffee can sustain you for hours without eating. However, for those who are fasting, coffee may become a double-edged sword. As you drink more and more coffee, you can gain a temporary respite and support to continue fasting. However, as you continue with this routine, you may end up developing a dependence on coffee, and that becomes unhealthy. Too much coffee can disrupt your sleeping cycle which can cause anxiety, even depression. For those who are already suffering from these conditions, this can be a fatal mistake. It can also boost cortisol production which can elevate your sugar level and develop insulin resistance.

You can develop food intolerance and risk of inflammation.

Your body is used to taking regular meals. When you fast, you are essentially disrupting the routine that your body has been used to. With this disruption, your body will need to adjust, and, in this transition, you will experience cravings for food. To satisfy these cravings, you will end up eating more. You won't be satisfied with just a slice of pizza or just a bite of donut, you may end up eating more along with reactive products like gluten foods, dairy products, and more. This abrupt onslaught of reactive foods may result to leaky gut, food intolerance, or inflammation.

You can develop eating disorders.

Perhaps the greatest risk that intermittent fasting can deliver is the development of eating disorders. Since intermittent fasting will lead you to skip meals in a row, the next time you eat, you may end up binge eating on your next meal. This continuous pattern of eating and not eating can warp into an eating disorder like bulimia, anorexia nervosa, and other eating disorders. To those who are already suffering from eating disorders, this can be a fatal mistake.

Intermittent Fasting: Men VS Women

Men and women have different responses when it comes to lifestyle changes, especially eating patterns or specific diets. Generally, men have the better adaptability to these changes than women this is because the effects of these changes take a while to take effect and by the time they do take effect, the body has already adapted. For women, the effects of these changes vary. Some women can go through the changes brought about by intermittent fasting with nothing but a minor bout of discomfort, usually for the first couple of days. After that, it's as if nothing happened and they are left with the bodies they dreamed of. However, there are also some who end up with more losses than gains. Some women cannot easily adapt to the change, so they end up developing adrenal issues, pregnancy issues, hormonal issues, and more.

This is the main reason why, as a woman, if you want to engage in fasting, it is better to start with short periods first and work your way up to slowly and gradually build up your body. Fasting at for 12 hours and eating within 12 hours is a good start. You can up the cycle to 14/10 after a few weeks. Men can start with 14/10 or 16/8 cycle and move up from there since the male body adapts faster to sudden changes than female bodies.

It is also recommended that to counter the effects of skipped meals, the meals taken during the eating hours should be nutrient-dense and not just a bag of junk. Some examples are water, black coffee, non-caloric drinks, banana, seeds and nuts, whole grains, and more. Munching or drinking these treats during fasting window will help curb your hunger. It is also highly recommended to be cautious as you proceed with your plans. Avoid fasting for too long as it can affect hormonal balance and related aspects.

Chapter 2: Positive Effects of Intermittent Fasting

Intermittent fasting affects many aspects of the body. However, the main targets are centered on hormonal balance, better metabolism, longevity, and more. Below are the top 6 beneficiaries of intermittent fasting:

Intermittent Fasting and Hormones

A lot of skeptics have questioned the impact of intermittent fasting on hormonal balance. There are some who dwells on the negative impact of fasting on the hormonal balance of women, while some focus more on the healing and balancing effects of the method.

Interestingly, fasting affects the female hormones more than the males'. Research has found out that when done correctly, fasting can stimulate the kisspeptin, protein used for communication between neurons, of the body which is essential in the maintenance of the GnRH. Fasting is also known to increase the secretion of the growth hormone which can do wonders to the muscles, tissues, and more.

Intermittent Fasting and Insulin Resistance

It is important to take note that intermittent fasting is a total body exercise package. Another benefit that it can bring is its impact on lowering insulin levels as well as insulin resistance. Sometimes, problems occur where the body does not respond to the insulin produced, leading to insulin resistance.

Insulin is released by the pancreas and it travels the body via the bloodstream. The cells of the body read the signal from insulin to utilize the sugar in the blood. If insulin resistance occurs, the body will refuse to read the signal emitted by insulin and will lead to the build-up of sugar in the blood resulting from diabetes. Fasting can help manage the amount of sugar in the blood by stimulating the production of insulin and the body's sensitivity to the protein, minimizing the possibility of developing insulin resistance.

Intermittent Fasting and Better Metabolism

The research found out that intermittent fasting is indeed beneficial to one's metabolism. Intermittent fasting helps burn the fat in the body without jeopardizing lean body mass. Most diet fads out there promotes burning of fat to lose weight. However, along with the process, lean body mass is also lost.

Intermittent fasting ensures that there is as less amount possible of lean body mass that is lost while converting fat to be more metabolically active and better at burning more calories.

Intermittent Fasting and Longevity

For centuries, people have studied different methods in order to increase the lifespan. A lot of vitamins and other supplements have been created in order to increase the vitality of cells to help the body endure longer. People have focused on medicines and medications so much that they neglect to consider the very simple and less expensive way of increasing longevity through intermittent fasting.

According to recent studies, intermittent fasting can, in fact, increase the lifespan of a person. Intermittent fasting alters the activities of the mitochondrial networks within cells that can slow down cellular aging and increase their lifespan. Through fasting, these mitochondrial networks are put under a restricted diet which promotes homeostasis. To adapt the restriction, the cells increase the plasticity of the fused and fragmented parts of the network. With preserving the homeostasis of these networks, the longevity and health of the cells will be increased.

Intermittent Fasting and Healthier Skin

In today's world, women often get hyped when there are new trends that can give them younger-looking and healthier skin. This is because a healthy glowing skin often reflects youthfulness and beauty.

Intermittent fasting can help you improve the health of your skin. When you give your body a break to relax from digesting food and detoxifying itself, it actually prevents pimples and acne from breaking out. Fasting can help the body focus on cleaning itself rather than on digesting and processing food. Through cleaning, the dead cells are removed and the production of new cells are boosted, giving you fresher and younger skin.

Intermittent Fasting and Losing Weight

Essentially, when you fast, you are actually consuming fewer calories than usual. Since the body receives fewer calories, it will use the fat stored in your body as the source of energy. As your body burn that fat for energy, you will eventually lose weight.

Intermittent fasting helps increase the level of HGH in your body as well as insulin. Human Growth Hormone (HGH) helps boost your body's fat burning capability to better harness energy from your stored fats.

This is also true for insulin. Fasting can help control the level of insulin in your blood. Insulin helps your body lose the excess fat and keep them from coming back. When you eat foods with processed carbohydrates like pasta, bread, rice, and the like, your insulin levels suddenly spike and then crash back down. To keep up with these sudden changes, your body will keep the food that you eat as fat instead of using them for energy. Fasting removes this problem.

Chapter 3: Methods of Intermittent Fasting for Women

Intermittent Fasting for Women: Results to Expect

Women who undergo intermittent fasting can experience different benefits and results. This is because although intermittent fasting offers several benefits, it still depends on the body on how to accept the change and to the person on how they go about with doing intermittent fasting. However, when done correctly, here are some of the results of intermittent fasting that you can expect:

Better metabolism.

When you do intermittent fasting right, one of the things that you can expect as a great result is better metabolism. However, it is important to note that fasting can be a wild card when it comes to increasing or slowing down metabolism. If you skip meals for too long, your body will adapt to the prolonged hunger by slowing down your metabolism. But, if you fast for short-periods only, as with intermittent fasting, your body will adapt by increasing your metabolism.

Shedding off a few pounds.

Fasting can lead to significant weight loss if it is done correctly. Just be careful when aiming for weight loss exclusively with intermittent fasting though. If your main goal of fasting is to lose weight and you end up at a weight plateau after the fasting period, you are setting yourself up for disappointment. So, instead of for aiming to lose weight, aim to improve your general well-being. As you proceed to make yourself healthier, weight loss will become easier for you.

Dewy and healthier skin.

Another result that you can expect out of intermittent fasting is healthier skin. Intermittent fasting helps your body clean itself. One of the best side effects is that your dead cells get cleaned as well leaving behind younger and healthier cells for your skin. With healthier skin, you can avoid acne and pimple breakouts.

Reduce the risk of diabetes.

The decrease in the risks of developing diabetes is another result that you can expect from fasting. When you fast, you are decreasing the amount of calorie that you take in. Since most calories that you take comes from processed sugars and carbs, regularly eat these foods can increase your risk of developing diabetes. However, by cutting your intake of such foods, you reduce the risks of diabetes.

Decrease risk of cardiovascular diseases.

When you lose weight because of intermittent fasting, it means that your body has burned the excess fat that is stored in your arteries, cells, etc. These fats are the main reasons why you can be at risk of developing cardiovascular diseases. However, with them gone, your chances of developing such diseases significantly decreases.

Although intermittent fasting is a widespread concept, there are still a few variations on how people apply it in their daily life. These variations are patterned on several factors, mainly on the variation of fasting and eating time. Some of the most popular methods out there today are:

The Crescendo Method

Compared to men, women are more sensitive to fluctuations in hunger. Hence, fasting for an entire week without any break is usually not advised. To cope with this need while still being able to apply intermittent fasting is the main focus of crescendo fasting.

As one of the more popular methods of the bunch, crescendo fasting is done by choosing non-consecutive days of the week as fasting days and the other non-consecutive days as normal eating days. Fasting hours are also between 12 to 16 hours and not more.

Essentially, with a crescendo, you can choose two to three non-consecutive days to fast for 12 to 16 hours. The remaining interval days, you will eat normally. For example, you choose to fast every Tuesday, Thursday, and Saturday for 14 hours. You can stop eating at 6 PM and resume a regular eating routine at 8 AM. On the other half of the days, you resume your normal eating routine.

When you fast with the crescendo, you get to fast for shorter periods which will still help you lose those extra calories. Furthermore, you don't have to worry about your sudden change in eating habit affecting your hormones and causing unfavorable changes.

The 16/8 Method

As the name suggests, the 16/8 method entails a fasting-eating cycle of 16 hours to 8 hours. It means that you reserve 16 hours of your day as fasting time and you will only restrict your eating time to 8 hours. For example, you can fast starting at 6 PM, Monday and eat your first meal at 10 AM, Tuesday.

The hours might be long, but within the 16-hour fasting window, you can consume tea, black coffee, sparkling water, diet sodas, and other similar beverages. After this fasting time, your 8-hour eating time can be filled with eating whatever you're like.

However, it is important to note though that since the 16/8 method is not a progressive type of fasting, unlike crescendo. Hence, you can do this every day of the week. Although it can potentially give you more visible results when it comes to losing weight, there is also a higher risk that your body may not be able to adjust quickly which may affect your hormones, causing delayed menstruation, etc.

This type of eating pattern may also be harder to maintain and needs commitment which is why is mostly recommended for those people who are used to skipping meals at long periods. These are mostly women who are so busy at work, usually arriving too late, that they forgo food for sleep. The body has already been used to the routine and has adapted which makes the 16/8 method not that far-fetched.

The 5:2 Diet

Some people are not so keen on watching the hours when they are supposed to stop eating and when they should resume eating. Some are more intuned with the days. Hence, people who enter into the intermittent fasting pool dive right into the 5:2 Diet pattern.

In the 5:2 diet, instead of minding the hours, you are actually minding the days. In this method, you have 5 days of the week where you eat normally. The remaining two days, you fast. However, it does not mean though that when you "fast" in these days, you eat nothing. No, simply, you eat about a quarter of what you usually eat. Women are advised to eat no more than 500 calories and men at 600 calories for the entire day. Hence, loading on vegetables, fishes, eggs, and other foods with the highest hunger satiation ability but with the least amount of calories are advised.

It is also recommended to choose non-consecutive fasting days, meaning you can eat normally on Mondays, Tuesdays, Thursdays, and Fridays, and fast on

Wednesday and Saturday. This is so that you give your body a break between eating and fasting.

In this method, you won't have to worry about non-eating hours. Just mind about eating less on your chosen fasting days and you'll be good to go. You are losing extra calories while not halting your eating regimen, simply toning it down a few notches.

The 24-Hour Protocol

Essentially, as what the name of the method implies, if you decide to apply this method, you will spend a full 24 hours fasting. This method is also known as the Eat-Fast-Eat method. This intermittent fasting method covers assigning one or two days in a week to fast for 24 hours. It could be that you eat your last meal at 8 PM Tuesday and supplement your stomach for the rest of the time with black coffee, water or tea. You then, eat your next meal on Wednesday at 8 PM. You can then repeat this on Saturday night as your last eating time and Sunday night to have your first meal after fasting.

Some people eat a heavy meal at the start of their 24-hour fast and end their fast with a simple snack. There is really no specification on how you start or end your 24-hour fast. The important thing here is that you achieve the 24-hours. Just remember that within this 24 hours of not eating, you will feel hungry and that within this time, you should commit yourself to drink calorie-free beverages, water is best. You can also drink 2-3 cups of tea or black coffee.

This method is not recommended for those people who cannot survive a day without any solid food. It is also advised that you start your 24-hour fast during your busy hours, like work lunch or working hours, where you can't really think of food because you are busy working.

The Alternate-Day Fasting

The Alternate-Day Fasting method is also popularly known as the UpDayDownDay Diet, and as the name suggests, it means that you alternate between fasting and eating. The days that you eat normally are your Up days while the days you fast are your Down days. Your "Up" days can be the first, third, fifth, and seventh day or the week, while your "Down" days can be the on the second, fourth, and sixth day. During your Up days, you eat normally with no changes in your meals. But on your Down days, you can eat only a quarter or less of what you normally eat.

However, there are also those who do a complete fast on the Down days, meaning there is no meal at all, only water, tea or black coffee. Now, although this one is doable, it is not advised for women who are still new to intermittent fasting. This is because going food-free for three days of the week can have repercussions for one's health, especially on those sensitive hormones.

Hence, if you wish to try out this fasting method, it is best to still have meals on your Down days. Just make sure to keep them below 400 or 500 calories.

The Warrior Diet

The concept of the Warrior Diet can be traced back to the eating regimens of warriors. Warriors of long ago spent the better part of the day training. They only get to eat and rest after training, at night. The training usually takes the better part of 20 hours and the remaining 4 hours is spent resting and eating.

Applied today, this method focuses on undereating and promoting eating at night. Eating is done at night because it delves into the nature of people as nocturnal eaters. However, it does not mean that throughout the entire 20 hours of fasting, you are not allowed to consume anything. You can eat fresh fruits, vegetables, and non-caloric drinks. These fasting meals are for maximizing the "fight or flight" response of the nervous system to boost energy, enhance metabolism, and promote alertness during the day.

When the fast ends, it is advised that for the one heavy meal you will eat within the 4-hour eating window, you prioritize eating vegetables, proteins, and fat. If you are still not full enough after the meal, that is the only time that you can eat carbohydrates. This limited eating will help boost digestion, relax and calm the body, and help it heal from the day's strenuous activities.

The Spontaneous Meal Skipping

If you are someone who is not keen on following any routine, then the other methods may not be for you. However, that does not mean that you cannot do intermittent fasting. You don't really have to follow a fixed eating-fasting cycle in order to engage in intermittent fasting. By simply skipping some meals every now and then, you are still doing some fasting.

Provided that it may not be as intensive as the other methods, spontaneous meal skipping can still deliver good results. If you are not really up to eating breakfast on any day, you can skip that meal and eat a healthy meal for lunch and dinner. The good thing about spontaneous skipping is that you fast whenever you want to. This is good for those who are far too busy at work that they unintentionally forget to eat. If you are too busy to eat lunch because of work, skip. If you are not really hungry, then you don't really have any reason to eat, unless you are following a strict medical routine.

You can even choose to skip two meals a day, usually breakfast and dinner, especially if you have a very hectic schedule for the day. Just make sure that you eat a healthy one for your next meal.

Whichever intermittent fasting method that takes your fancy, just make sure that it is the one that will work best for you. It is not recommended that you rush through any method without thinking it and even consulting experts if further support is required.

Remember that before you engage in any intermittent fasting regimen, your health and general well-being must always come first.

Chapter 4: Intermittent Fasting and Body Awareness

It is important that for women, like you, engaging in intermittent fasting is not done abruptly and whimsically. If you decide to engage in intermittent fasting, you must be sure of your willingness to commit and be prepared to deal with the changes, both good and bad. This is the very reason why you must learn and consider your personal aims, goals, physical state, and other important factors first.

Listening to the Body and Its Needs

Some women who indulge in intermittent fasting do so haphazardly. They do it to achieve their goal, primarily to lose weight. They do it despite the screams and warning signs of their body which should not be the case. Remember, before you decide to engage in any activity that could have a significant effect on your body, always prioritize your health. What is the use of achieving the perfect beach body when end up suffering end the end? So, always consider your health first.

Now, there are a lot of things that your body needs that you must achieve while still being able to intermittent fasting. Here are the top concerns:

Do not neglect your nutrition.

When you engage in intermittent fasting, it is a given that you will be removing some calories. However, that does not mean that you also cut on the nutrition. There are a lot of ways on how you can augment the loss of calories by eating healthy meals packed with vegetables, fruits, lean meats and non-caloric drinks on your meals. Do not sacrifice nutrition for weight loss. You will still lose those extra calories without having to cut on your needed nutritional values.

Ease into the method.

As a woman, your body reacts differently to changes compared to men. Hence, it is important that when you engage in intermittent fasting, especially if it is your first time, you do things gradually. Do not engage in a full-out fast immediately like the Warrior Diet, or the 24-Hour Protocol. You can try those after you get the hang of things. It is better to start with the milder methods first like the Crescendo Method, the 16/8 Method, or the 5:2 Diet. If these methods are still too abrupt for you, just go with the basic Spontaneous Meal Skipping.

Stay hydrated.

Your body needs water to function properly. It is important that while you do intermittent fasting, you always stay hydrated. You can drink water, tea, black coffee, and other non-calorie drinks. These types of drinks will keep you well-hydrated without impending on your intermittent fasting plans.

Intermittent Fasting: Following VS Understanding

One of the main problems with women who engage in intermittent fasting is that those who are completely new to the trend end up just following steps without fully understanding the entire method. This leads to many consequences throughout the entire processes. Therefore, it is very important to not just follow whatever intermittent fasting process you might want to try out but to understand how to do intermittent fasting properly.

When you engage in intermittent fasting, you must understand the entire process to be able to identify which portions of the method will not work for you. For example, you want to try out the 24-hour Protocol because a friend did it and you think that it will give you the fastest trim down you need to get your dream bikini body. However, you have never tried fasting for the same length or even half the time before. When you try out the method, you may end up inflicting pain on yourself more than helping.

This goes back to how important it is to understand your body's needs first. Before you engage in any intermittent fasting method, you must have a full understanding of what you should and should not do, and what you should and should not have. Getting a clear understanding of what you want to achieve, how you will achieve those goals, and what are the things to consider before you begin, will help ease out the kinks of the process. It will infinitesimally make your life easier and healthier.

So, once again, remember that you don't have to follow every single step and trend in the intermittent fasting verse. What is important here is that you fully understand the risks, the benefits, and the ways on how you can help yourself ease in to and adapt to the change.

Chapter 5: Your Food Choices and Intermittent Fasting

One of the biggest problems when it comes to intermittent fasting is not knowing which foods you can eat throughout the phase, and which you should stay miles away from. As a woman, sometimes it takes a lot of commitment and discipline to stay away from your favorite comfort food, especially when it is filled with all those calorie goodness. It is also quite difficult to identify which foods are passable enough to eat, which are necessary to eat, and which you should completely avoid while doing intermittent fasting. Hence, this chapter will cater to that particular concern.

The Right Food to Eat

Aside from sticking to your fasting hours, eating the right foods during your eating hours is also important. Even though there are no restrictions on what you can eat on your eating window, some necessary limitations will still be better. For example, you fast for 14 hours, and then you load on burgers, fries, beers, and all those carbs-rich foods during your 10-hour eating window. Imagine, will the fasting actually work this way? No, right! It is because to get the best possible result for you when you do intermittent fasting, it is still better to eat foods that will actually boost the effects and not impede them.

So, what foods and beverages should you consume during your eating window? Well, here are the top 10:

Water

It is very important that when you are doing intermittent fasting, you always keep yourself hydrated.

To do that, you must binge on water. You can drink other non-calorie drinks. However, water is still the best. It keeps your organs healthy and keeps you well-hydrated. If you cannot stomach, drinking just pure water throughout the entire ordeal, you can squeeze in lemon juice to give it a bit of a kick. Also, remember the important signs of dehydration. When your urine turns dark yellow, it means you are dehydrated. The paler the color of the urine is the better your health is, so you must drink lots of water.

Whole Grains

Eating lots of carbs is a big violation of the entire concept of intermittent fasting. However, it does not mean that you should avoid it altogether. You can still enjoy a few carbs through consuming whole grains. These grains have high fiber content as well as rich in protein.

This means that even with eating small portions, you will still full which will lessen your urge to eat. Studies also show that whole grains can increase your metabolism, which is highly valuable when fasting.

Avocados

Avocado is known to be a high-calorie fruit. However, because most of the fat in the avocado is monounsaturated, it gives you higher satiation. Many studies show that adding avocados in your meal during fasting will keep you full longer than when you are eating these delicious fruits. You also don't have to eat the entire fruit to be full. All you need is half the portion mixed with your meal, and you can go long hours without feeling hungry.

Fish

If you plan to fast, it is important that you include fish in your next meal. This is because is known to be rich in protein and healthy fats. There are also high amounts of vitamins, particularly Vitamin D. Since your aim by fasting is to each less food than you usually do, why not choose one that is packed with high nutritional value? It also adds to the sweet deal that fish can help boost your mental health without impeding your body goals.

Fiber-rich foods

Whether you go on a diet, a strict regimen for fasting, or any food trend, it is quite common to hear advertisements left and right pushing people to eat fiber-rich foods. This is because fiber-rich foods like brussels sprouts, broccoli, cauliflower, and more help stabilize your bowels. These foods help you avoid getting constipation throughout your fasting journey and they also help in keeping you full for longer hours which is essential if you want to avoid binge eating after your fasting window.

Beans and Legumes

Carbs restriction is not really that strict if you plan to do intermittent fasting. However, since women can gain significant weight when lots of carbohydrates are introduced into the routine, it is best to stick to limited amounts. One of the best foods to eat to still get carbs but at low amounts are beans like chickpeas, lentils, and other legumes. Beans and legumes are also known to be great at boosting weight loss even if you are not reigning in those calories.

Eggs

Eggs are a very well-known staple food for some travelers. This is because eggs are packed with lots of proteins and takes less time to cook than say, rice and other foods which makes great for long hours without eating. Because they contain lots of proteins, about 6 grams for large ones, you will be less hungry when you eat eggs and can go longer without food. This very nature of eggs makes them an ideal food for intermittent fasting.

Nuts

If you feel hungry while you are fasting, why not chump on some nuts. Although they have higher calories than other snacks you can eat, nuts are high in polyunsaturated fats which are great for dampening your hunger urges and gives longer satiety. Walnuts and almonds are great examples. Whenever you feel that your meal is not enough to make you last longer, instead of piling in more food, why not eat some walnuts, almonds, hazel, or some other nuts instead.

Berries

Smoothies are very common for those in a diet, doing intermittent fasting is no different. Smoothies are commonly made from fruits and vegetables. Some of the most popular ingredients are berries like strawberries, blueberries, and cranberries. Berries are packed with vitamin C which is vital for your immune system. One cup of berries thrown in on your smoothie or eaten raw accumulates over 100 percent of the required daily value. Berries are also rich in flavonoids which are known to slow down weight gain, as studies have shown.

Probiotic-rich foods

Your stomach has tiny natural inhabitants that when upset when the balance is changed. When you do intermittent fasting, you can expect your eating routine to diverge from what you are used to. This upsets the balance in your stomach which in turn, also upsets those little critters causing irritation that can lead to constipation, among other side effects. To help counter these effects, it is recommended to load on probiotics. Foods rich in probiotics such as yogurt, kraut, kombucha, pickles, kimchi, miso, kefir, and others should be a staple in your fasting meals.

Foods to Avoid

If there are "a-must" foods in your menu, then there are also "a-must-avoid" ones. These must-avoid foods can impede and dampen the effects of fasting. This is the reason why that if you can refrain from adding them in your meals, then do so, but if they cannot be avoided, then consume them by small amounts only and as much as possible, eating two or more of them together. So, here are the top 10 foods you can definitely do away within your meals:

White Rice

Carbs are your greatest enemy when you are fasting. Hence, indulging in rice while doing so is a big no. This is because rice, especially the white variety, contains high amounts of starch, and starch is the storage medium of carbs. When you eat white rice for your meal right after your fast, it will cause adverse effects like lethargy or drowsiness. White rice is also easily stored as fat which promotes weight gain.

Fried Foods

Fried foods are also some of the foods that you must avoid right after you finish fasting. This is because fried foods are filled with saturated fats and other excess fats. Usually, when you have your first meal after the fasting period, it is highly possible that you will binge on the food. If you binge on fried food, this will lead to more fat being stored in your body, leading to weight gain. This greatly defeats the purpose of fasting.

Carbonated Drinks

Carbonated drinks have high sugar content. Lots of sugar in your meal right after fasting will only cause you to be lethargic and less active. Carbonated drinks will also shock your stomach from the sudden onslaught of sugar which may lead to constipation, flatulence, and other possible problems. If you feel thirsty while eating your meal, drink cold water instead or some tea.

Coffee

Although it is sometimes advised to drink coffee while you are fasting to control your hunger, there are some other disadvantages to them as well. Consuming coffee without any food during fasting will only cause the acid in your gut to rise, making you sick. If you are fond of drinking a cup or two of coffee, make sure you drink black coffee only with no sugar, cream or milk added because it will be easier on the stomach and always eat something along with it.

Fatty Foods

Consuming foods with too much fat right after fasting or while fasting is not recommended. This is because these foods will only add to the fat stored in your body leading to more calories, something that you should be burning in the first place. If you really need some fats in you to keep you satisfied while fasting, why don't you feast on some nuts like walnuts instead?

Refined Sugar

Consuming products mixed with refined sugars can detrimental to the effects of fasting. Whenever you get hungry right after a fast, it is recommended to avoid eating sweet foods such as bagels, ice cream, chocolates, and other desserts immediately. This is because even when you are fasting, your body will be able to utilize all those sugars in time, some of them will only be stored as part of excess fat which will contribute to weight gain.

White Flour

White flour is also a must-avoid when fasting. This is because white flour has already been processed and stripped of the essential fibers that can help improve the condition of your bowels. Products made of white flour, such as bread are also nothing much but empty calories. They no longer have the essential nutrients that are important to keep you healthy. Instead of eating foods made of white flour such as regular bread, cereals, crackers, go for whole grains instead. There are varieties of whole grain bread and crackers available in the market to satiate your needs.

Preserved Foods

Preserved foods or foods that have been pre-packed in sold un markets contain preservatives and artificial ingredients that are not good for your body.

Even while you are not fasting, it is always best to go organic. Instead of eating tomatoes out of the can, try to take time to buy some fresh produce instead. These preserved foods will only satisfy your momentarily and will immediately make you hungry again.

Salty Foods

Consuming salty products right after going for hours without food can only cause problems for you. Salty foods can increase your blood pressure causing you to feel sick. It can also cause an upset stomach due to the sudden onslaught of salt in your gut. Hence, as much as possible, avoid eating salty foods when you are fasting. If it really cannot be helped, always drink water first and eat small portions at a time only.

Dairy Products

Dairy products are such great temptations right after a fast. However, remember that your stomach is rather sensitive after having been dormant for hours during your fast and may not be able to suggest foods with large calorie content immediately. Hence, it is important that you don't consume foods with lots of calories immediately because it will only harm your stomach causing constipation and stomach ache. Milk and other dairy products are packed with lots of calories so as much as possible, refrain from eating them while you are doing intermittent fasting.

It is important to stay vigilant and aware of the foods that you eat when you are doing intermittent fasting. This is because if you are not closely monitoring what you are eating, you may end up derailing your progress. Instead of losing those extra calories, you might end up gaining more than what you are shedding which is the opposite of what fasting should be.

How to Schedule Meals: Intermittent Fasting for Beginners

When to schedule your meals is an essential aspect of intermittent fasting. For women, it is important that you schedule your meals strategically in order to avoid as much change in your body that can affect the hormonal balance of your body. If you are unsure about how to proceed it is always recommended to consult your doctor first.

Anyways, if you have already set your mind and is eager to jumpstart your intermittent fasting journey, here is a break down of a simple meal schedule that you can follow. The meal plan is broken down into three:

beginner, intermediate, upper intermediate, and advanced.

Beginner Plan

If you are a beginner to intermittent fasting, then it is important to keep things simple and easy. For starters, you can have you fasting window at hours that are more convenient for you. You can start your fast from 6 PM until 8 AM the next day and your eating window from 8 AM to 6 PM. That will give you 14-hours of fasting time, and 10-hours eating time. Having a schedule such as this will help you gradually adjust to long hours of not eating while not missing three meals a day. You can even munch on some small snacks with your meals.

You can follow this pattern:

8:00 – Breakfast

12:00 – Lunch

2:30 – Snacks

6:00 – Dinner

You can choose to do this every day, but as a beginner, it is recommended to do this moderately so doing this for 2-3 days a week can a good start. Do not immediately jump into the fray. Make your body adjust to the changes first.

Intermediate Plan

If you are not a complete newbie to intermittent fasting but is still hesitant to go for long hours, then the intermediate plan is for you. With this schedule, you can have 16 hours of fasting time and 8 hours of eating time. You can also rev it up a bit by going for 18 hours fasting and 6 hours of eating. You have longer hours for fast but not too long that will shock your body immediately. You must also only engage in this type of plan if you have tried intermittent fasting already.

For the 16-8 plan, you can follow this schedule:

10:00 – Snacks / Small meal

12:00 – Lunch

2:30 – Snack

6:00 – Dinner

For the 18-6 plan, you can follow this schedule:

12:00 – Lunch

2:30 – Snack

6:00 – Dinner

It is at your discretion whether you plan to do this daily or at selected days of the week only. If you are not completely sure about what to do, you can follow this meal plan 2-3, even 4, days a week. This way you have days where you can eat normally and days where you can fast. Even when you are fasting daily, there are still days where you cut your calories consumption. That is still a huge cut out of your usual calorie intake per week.

Upper Intermediate Plan

If you feel more confident with intermittent fasting, you can go higher with the upper intermediate plan. In this plan, you can select two non-consecutive days of the week to eat nothing and consume fluids only. The remaining 5 days, you can eat normal meals.

Here is a sample plan for the 2 days where you will fast for 24 hours:

Tuesday

7:00 PM – Last meal with water

Wednesday

7:00 AM – No meal, drink water or tea

12:00 PM – No meal, drink water or tea

3:00 PM – No meal, drink water or tea

7:00 – Fast Ends, eat a small dinner with lots of organic carbs like whole grains, good protein from beans and legumes or lean meat, and water.

Repeat this schedule again on Friday or Saturday.

Only follow this plan if you are sure you can take a full 24-hours without solid food. If you think you cannot do this or if your doctor advises you against it, then, by all means, do not proceed. Always prioritize your health over losing weight or whatever purpose you may have for fasting.

Advanced Plan

In this schedule, you will go for alternate days of fasting. The time breakdown is the same with the Upper Intermediate plan. The only difference is that with that plan you will only for 2 non-consecutive days without eating food. On this plan, you will do for every other day without food.

For example, on day 1 you do a 24-hour fast, then eat normal meals on day 2. Day 3 is another fast day while day 4 is your normal eating day. Day 5 and day 6 follows the same pattern. Day 7 can also be a normal eating day to give yourself a reprieve from fasting.

For the days that you are eating normally, load yourself on clean meats, fruits and vegetables, healthy fats from beans, and other healthy food. Refrain from consuming empty calories which can disrupt the entire process.

Only engage in this type of schedule if you have been intermittently fasting for some time and wants to go higher. If you have never tried going without food for days a week, then this is not recommended for you. No matter how desperate you are to achieve that bikini body, it is not worth the hype if you end up collapsing. This is the most intense plan that not all can safely do, but when done properly and safely, this gives astonishing results.

Chapter 6: Sample Recipes for Intermittent Fasting

Deciding what to eat while doing intermittent fasting can be quite difficult which is why this chapter is dedicated to providing you with some good recipes to try out during your meals.

Breakfast

For breakfast, the idea is to keep your meals simple but packed with nutrients. Here are three recipes you can try:

Toast topped with Chia seeds, peanut butter, and banana

This twist from the classic Peanut butter and jelly toast is a great breakfast combo you can try with just 210 calories to burn.

Ingredients:

2 slices whole grain bread

1 tbsp. peanut butter

½ banana, sliced

½ tbsp. chia seeds

Procedure:

1. Toast the bread slices and then, spread the peanut butter on both slices.

2. Top each with sliced bananas and then, drizzle the chia seeds on top.

3. You can also add in a dash of cinnamon for added taste.

Egg and avocado toast

Here is another toast recipe that you will surely like. Toast a slice of whole grain bread, then top with mashed avocado and sunny-side up egg. This contains about 275 calories.

Ingredients:

1 slice of whole grain bread

1 oz of avocado

1 egg

salt and pepper

Procedure:

1.   First, toast the bread and then set aside.

2.   Mash the avocado in a bowl. Add salt and pepper to taste and set aside.

3.   On a pan, drizzle some oil and the fry the egg, sunny side up, to your liking.

4. Spread the mashed avocado on the toast and top with the sunny side up egg.

5. Add salt and pepper. You can also add hot sauce or regular tomato ketchup as well.

Yogurt, banana and berries smoothie

If munching on solid foods is not your ideal breakfast meal, then this yogurt and berries smoothie is a great alternative. This is ideal for those mornings when you are in a rush and don't have enough time to cook meals. You can even pre-blend this the night before and place it in the freezer as ready-to-go breakfast on your way to work. Using water gives about 190 calories. If you add low-fat milk instead of water, this raises to about 250 calories.

Ingredients:

1 cup Greek yogurt

1 ripe banana (medium), slice into chunks

1 cup water or low-fat milk

1 cup mixed berries (strawberry, blueberries, cranberries)

Procedures:

1. Combine all the ingredients in a blender and blend until smooth.

2. Pour on a tall glass, and then serve.

Lunch

Here are three easy-to-make lunch ideas that you can enjoy. The idea for lunch meals is to keep them packed with protein, vitamins, and minerals, without going overboard.

Black beans and avocado burrito

This simple burrito recipe is a great meal choice for lunch on the go. The beans are great sources of fiber and the avocado is high on monounsaturated fats. This meal packs 365 calories

Ingredients:

1 whole wheat burrito wrap

¼ cup black beans

2 or 3 slices of avocados

¼ cup sliced onions (optional)

Hot sauce (optional)

Procedures:

1. In a pan, toast the whole wheat burrito until desired crispiness. Set aside.

2. Pan fry the black beans or cook in the microwave.

3. Slice the avocado into ½ thick slices. You can use 2 or more slices.

4. Get the burrito wrap. Fill with the black beans and top with the sliced avocados. You can also add some sliced onions and a drizzle of hot sauce for extra kick.

Chicken and cheese sandwich

If meat is your must-have during lunch, then try this chicken and cheese sandwich recipe. This total to about 395 calories.

Ingredients:

2 slices whole wheat bread

½ slice chicken breast

1 lettuce leaf

1 slice Swiss cheese

2 tbsp. Low-fat mayonnaise

2 slices of tomatoes

Procedures:

1. Grill the chicken breast to desired finish.

2. Spread the mayonnaise on both whole wheat bread slices.

3. Layer the lettuce leaf on one of the slices.

4. Place the grilled chicken on top of the lettuce.

5. Top with the Swiss cheese and sliced tomatoes.

Garden salad and pasta mix

If pasta and salads are your things, then this recipe is great for you. The key player in this dish is to use whole-grain pasta instead of the regular ones. This contains about 400 calories.

Ingredients:

1 pack whole grain pasta

1 cup shredded chicken breast

½ cup Parmesan cheese

½ cup carrots (sliced thinly)

½ cup green bell pepper

¼ cup chopped celery

1 cup cherry tomatoes

½ cup green onion (chopped)

¾ cup low-fat mayonnaise

2 tbsp. lemon juice

Procedures:

1.   Cook the pasta in boiling water until al dente. Rinse, drain and set aside.

2.   Pan fry chicken breast and shred.

3.   Mix the pasta, chicken breast, carrots, bell pepper, celery, tomatoes, and onions.

4.   Add in the mayonnaise and the lemon juice. Mix well.

5.   Chill before serving.

Snacks

Eating something in-between your meals is still possible even when you are fasting. Just make sure to keep your snacks simple and less in calories. Here are three great recipes:

Carrot and parmesan fries

One of the classic snacks there is is French fries. However, they are something you can do away while fasting. That does not mean though that you cannot eat something similar. Substitute the potato with sliced carrots instead. This simple snack is only around 85 calories.

Ingredients:

3 large carrots

¼ cup grated parmesan cheese

3 tbsp olive oil

½ tsp salt

¼ tsp pepper

1 tsp garlic powder

¼ cup mayonnaise

2 tsp lemon juice

Procedures:

1. Preheat the oven to 400 degrees Fahrenheit.

2. Peel and cut the carrots into fries.

3. In a bowl, mix the olive oil, garlic powder, salt, pepper, and parmesan cheese. Make sure to set aside a little of the garlic powder, salt and pepper for the dip.

4. Add the carrots to the mixture and mix well.

5. Bake the coated carrots for 15-20 minutes or until carrots become soft and slightly crispy. Don't forget to turn carrots halfway through.

6. In a separate container, mix the mayonnaise, lemon juice, garlic powder, salt and pepper to make the dip.

7. Once the carrot fries are cooked and cooled, serve with the dip.

Greens wrap

If you are strong on veggies, this snack is a great choice. You can take this on the go or eat on a plate. This meal is a great combo of recipes with about 115 calories.

Ingredients

1 large lettuce leaf

¼ cup hummus

½ cup thinly sliced carrots

½ cup thinly sliced cucumber (strips)

¼ cup green bell pepper

½ cup cherry tomatoes

2 or 3 slices avocado

Procedures:

1. Spread the lettuce leaf on a flat surface.

2. Spread hummus on the leaf with a 2-inches free as border.

3. Top the leaf with the carrots, cucumber, bell pepper, tomatoes, and avocado. Make sure to leave space at the sides for folding.

4. Fold the sides of the leaf towards the center and roll away from you, like a burrito.

5. Wrap it with plastic wrap and chill before serving.

Banana muffin with Nutella filling

Can you imagine eating a muffin with Nutella as snacks when you are doing intermittent fasting? Quite impossible, right? Well, now it's not. You easily make this dessert without having to worry about the calories with just 185 to burn.

Ingredients:

1 ¼ cup whole-wheat flour

2 scoops protein powder

½ cup non-fat Greek yogurt

1 tbsp ground flaxseeds

1/8 tsp salt

2 large eggs

2 tsp baking powder

¼ cup skim milk

2 ripe bananas mashed

1 tbsp vanilla extract

¼ cup Nutella

Procedures:

1. Preheat the oven to 350 degrees Fahrenheit.

2. Spray cooking oil or olive oil on a 12-cup muffin pan.

3. In a bowl, mix the whole wheat flour, protein powder, baking powder, flaxseeds, and salt.

4. In a separate bowl, combine the eggs, bananas, yogurt, skim milk, and vanilla extract.

5. Mix the dry and wet ingredients well.

6. Pour the mixture into the muffin cups halfway, then add a tsp of Nutella. Fill in the rest of the batter.

7. Bake for 18-20 minutes or until cooked through testing via toothpick method.

8. Cool and serve.

Dinner

Dinner is the last meal of the day. Most people skip this because they think that dinner meals are usually calorie-heavy. However, remember that dinner is as important as all the other meals. In fact, if you are doing a 24-hour fast, dinner is the most important meal of the day. Here are three meal ideas that you can try:

Stuffed bell peppers

This dinner meal is quite simple. Free of any grain with the same satisfaction, all with just 180 calories per bell pepper combo.

Ingredients:

3 bell peppers

3 large eggs

3 cups kale chopped

2 medium tomatoes chopped

½ tsp salt

½ tsp pepper

1 tsp thyme

1 tsp garlic powder

Procedures:

1.   Preheat oven to 400 degrees Fahrenheit.

2.   Cut the top of the bell peppers, remove the seeds and ribs without breaking the peppers. You can use the bell of your choice.

3.   Place the peppers in a muffin pan.

4.   Sauté the kale, tomatoes, and the top portion of the bell pepper over medium heat for 5 minutes or until kale is wilted. Add in salt to taste.

5.   In a separate bowl, combine the eggs, thyme and garlic powder. Season with salt and pepper to taste.

6.   Stuff the bell peppers with the combined veggies and the egg mixture. Be careful not to overfill. Then, bake for 30 minutes.

Roasted spiced salmon and cauliflower

Fish is a great choice for dinner. You can enjoy this recipe for your dinner with just 270 calories.

Ingredients:

4 salmon fillets (1 inch thick)

1 tbsp olive oil

1 tsp ground cumin

¾ tsp kosher salt

1/8 tsp ground black pepper

4 cups cauliflower florets

¼ cup chopped cilantro

¼ cup golden raisins

1 tbsp lemon juice

½ tsp ground coriander

1/8 tsp ground allspice

Procedures:

1. Preheat oven to 450 degrees Fahrenheit.

2. In a large bowl, combine the olive oil, ½ tsp cumin, ¼ tsp kosher salt, black pepper, and the cauliflower florets. Mix well.

3. Bake the cauliflower florets for 18-20 minutes or until tender and browned.

4. Once done, combine the florets with cilantro, lemon juice, and raisins. Toss well and set aside.

5. Reduce the temperature of the oven to 400 degrees.

6. In another bowl, combine allspice, the other ½ tsp of the cumin, and the remaining ½ tsp of kosher salt.

7. Rub the combined spices to the salmon fillets.

8. Bake the fillets at 400 degrees for 10-15 minutes or until cooked.

9.	Serve the florets and salmon together. Add in some lemon wedges for optional kick.

Classic pork with veggies

If you love pork, then this recipe is a classic. This packs around 458 calories which gives you satisfaction without dampening your fasting scheme.

Ingredients:

2 lbs. pork tenderloin

2 tbsp chopped rosemary

3 garlic cloves minced

1 tsp ground black pepper

1 1/8 tsp salt

4 tbsp olive oil

4 cups cauliflower florets

4 large carrots chopped

2 large green onions sliced

2 tsp Dijon mustard

1 ½ tsp maple syrup

Procedures:

1. Preheat oven to 400 degrees Fahrenheit.

2. In a bowl, mix the rosemary, garlic, salt, and pepper. Rub the mixture to the tenderloins.

3. Sear the tenderloin on all sides in a skillet over medium heat for 8-10 minutes. Then, transfer to the oven and cook for about 1 hour.

4. In a small bowl, mix Dijon mustard, olive oil, and maple syrup. Add in the cauliflower florets, onions, and carrots. Season with salt and pepper. Make sure toss the vegetable mixture well and roast until done.

5. Transfer the pork on a cutting board, cover with aluminum foil, and let is rest for 15 minutes. Slice the pork and serve with the roasted vegetables.

Chapter 7: Exercise and Intermittent Fasting

The Value of Exercise

Some women think that since they are engaging in intermittent fasting, there is no need to exert more effort to exercise since they are already losing the excess calories by fasting. They seem to forget that exercise is much more than just losing calories. Exercising is a form of maintaining the good functioning and condition of your body. It will help boost your metabolism and burn the carbs and fats away as energy. Aside from that, exercise also revitalizes your cells, giving you younger looking skin, and keep your mind active and healthy.

However, the big question now is that whether or not you can do exercise while doing intermittent fasting. Well, you still can. In fact, when you exercise while you are fasting burns more fats than when you eating normally. This is because when you eat normally, your body will burn all the carbs and calories first as a source of energy. When you cut your calories, your body will have to look for other sources of energy to sustain you, and the next viable source is the stored fats in your body. Studies show that women who exercise while fasting lost more calories than those who are not. Exercise can help boost the burning of fats to increase the rate of weight loss.

There is a catch though. Although exercising during fasting is a great help to enhance the effects of fasting, there is also a danger in that as well. If your body burns out the carbs and the fats as a source of energy, the next source available will be your protein reserves, the main building components of your muscles. While you may lose more fats and calories when exercising, there is also a risk of losing more muscles as well. When you exercise on an empty stomach, your body will eventually start breaking down the protein stored in your muscles for energy which will also deteriorate your muscles. Not only that, as you cut your daily calories, your body will adapt by slowing down your metabolism and burning lesser calories. This is to make sure that you do not overburn your energy and end up sick.

But, that does not mean that you should not exercise out of fear of the effects though. There are many ways on how you can tweak your exercises to match your intermittent fasting needs.

How to Exercise Safely During Intermittent Fasting

Remember that exercise is a very important component to keep you physically and mentally healthy. For those women out there who are absolute health buffs and are exercise geeks, there is still a safe way on how you can exercise while simultaneously cutting on your calorie intake by fasting. Here are some helpful tips that you can follow to get as much out of your workout without having to tip-toe around intermittent fasting:

Keep your cardio exercises low key when fasting.

When you do cardio workouts, refrain from doing extreme workouts that will cause you to burn energy fast. Remember that you are decreasing your calorie intake which means your energy levels will not be as high as those who are not fasting. So, keep your cardio workouts simple. Don't overexert yourself when a good light jog around the park will suffice. Gauge your breathing. If you can still talk normally while jogging, then good. However, when you feel dizzy or a bit light-headed, then you should stop. It is better to slow down than force yourself which will only do more harm than good.

Intensify the exercise only during the eating window or non-fasting days.

If you are planning to intensify your workout routine, do this only during your non-fasting hours or days. It is even recommended to schedule your workouts as close to your last meal as possible. This is because this is around this time that you have the most amount of carbs that serves as fuel for your body. Doing your exercise this way will also decrease your risk of suddenly dropping your sugar levels. You can also munch on some carb-rich snacks to provide more fuel for your muscles after your intense exercise since your muscles will still be buzzing for more energy around this time.

Indulge in lean protein to retain your muscles.

Remember that when your body runs out of carbohydrates to burn for energy, the next source will be fats, and when the fats are not enough, proteins will come next. Proteins are the main components of your muscles which means that as your body burns the proteins, your muscles will also slowly deteriorate. If you wish to retain your muscles while still burning off the extra pounds, you need to load on lean proteins. Hence, you must schedule your workouts, especially the strength-based ones, in-between two protein-rich meals. This will ensure that you have enough supply to burn away and enough left to repair your muscles.

Munch on snacks before and after a workout.

Most intermittent fasting methods give leeway for snack time. Make sure to take advantage of that to eat snacks that are rich in fast-acting carbs and proteins that are great sugar stabilizers. A great option is a whole grain toast topped with organic peanut butter and a slice of banana at the side. The importance of eating snacks before and after your workout is to ensure that you will not run out of energy source to burn during your exercise and for repairs after.

Who says exercise cannot be done while fasting? It is perfectly possible. All you need is proper planning and make sure to pattern your workouts around your meals to achieve the best results.

Chapter 8: Safeguarding Your Diet

How to Start Intermittent Fasting

For beginners, especially women, intermittent fasting can be very intimidating. This is because of the various information that litters the internet and the various claims of successes and failures. However, if you are completely new to intermittent fasting here are some simple steps that you can follow to jumpstart your journey:

Consult your doctor first.

Since this is your first time to do intermittent fasting, it is important that you talk to your doctor first. Ask for advice on which methods you can to minimize any possible effects on hour hormones and how to bounce back. You also need to clarify whether you are healthy enough to do intermittent fasting or not. Clearing these things out will help you decide whether you want to try out IF or not.

Define your purpose.

Once you receive the go signal to start fasting, you need to define next the purpose why you want to fast in the first place. Are you aiming to lose weight to wear that nice dress you saw at the mall? Are aiming to maintain your current weight? Do you want to improve your health in general? Whichever goal you want to achieve, just make sure that it is enough to keep you motivated and it is not too complicated that you end up dropping out in the middle of things.

Keep things simple and easy.

As a beginner, the best approach to start your fasting is to keep things simple and easy. Just because your friend is doing a full 18-hour fast doesn't mean that you should too. What is important is that you finish fast. Keep your food as healthy as possible. You also don't have to jump into cooking those super intricate recipes. Simple meals loaded with nutrients will do.

Time depends on you.

The time schedules listed in all those intermittent fasting manuals, even here, are just there as a reference. It doesn't mean that since it says dinner should be at 7 PM that you should eat at 7 PM. You can schedule your fasting and eating hours according to your convenience. This also applies to the days. There are no specific days to schedule your meals, those mentioned in the different methods are just guides. However, just remember that it is ideal if you can schedule you fasting hours or days during the days where you are so busy that you don't really keep tabs on your meals.

It's okay to slip up.

Don't push yourself too much. It is okay to slip up on your fasting. Perhaps that piece of glazed donut with fruity sprinkles on top is far too tempting to resist after a long fast. That's okay. When you slip up, don't quit. You can always do over. Just make sure to not repeat that slip up again. It will also help if you keep things simple that way you can minimize the slip-ups since things are not that complicated to follow through.

Tips and Tricks to Succeed in Intermittent Fasting

In the long run, you may find yourself exhausted and too tired to continue with fasting. Maybe the steps are too complicated or being hungry is just too much and the temptation to binge eat is just too much. Well, no worries. Here are some tips that can help stay on track:

Quitting? Visit your purpose.

Whenever you feel like quitting because maybe the effects are slow, or the hunger is too much, visit your goal again. Why are you doing intermittent fasting in the first place? Are you sure you want to be a wimp and just quit? Don't give up. A lot of women out there are willing to be on your shoes right now, so if they can commit enough to the deed, then why can't you?

Water is your ally.

Water can help you conquer the hunger. During your fasting window, drink lots of water. This will help you control your urge to eat. You need to be firm. Every time you think of eating before your supposed schedule, drink a cup of water instead.

Black coffee or tea.

If you think water too bland to supplement your hunger, go for black coffee and unsweetened tea instead. These two contains caffeine which can help tweedled down hour hunger. They are also zero-calorie drinks, so you don't have to worry about the possible carbs.

Be a busy bee.

Keep yourself busy. When you are busy thinking about work and other things, you will not think as much about eating. This is the main reason why it is best to schedule you fasting hours during your working hours since you'll be too busy to mind that scrumptious bag of bagel sitting on your colleague's desk, hopefully not yours.

Stay away from temptation.

Temptations are always everywhere. You need to keep control and stay away from them. If you sense your mother, friend, husband, etc. cooking a meal. Get yourself out of the house and go for a run. You won't only benefit from the exercise, but you also get to avoid the tempting smell of food being cooked. When you are invited to eat out, always keep in mind to order the healthy ones.

Eat wisely.

Since your meals are limited, you need to eat wisely. Instead of binge eating crappy foods like donuts, pizza, white rice, etc. for your next meal, eat fruits and vegetables, or lean meat instead. Choose foods that can give you the most nutritional value with the least number of calories. Be smart about what you are waiting.

Tone down your expectations.

Since you are still starting your intermittent fasting journey, you need to keep your expectations down low. Usually, the significant effects of intermittent fasting show around 2 to 3 weeks after starting. Don't expect too much, especially during the first weeks. Too much expectation will lead to greater disappointments and being disappointed in the results is one of the main precursors to quitting.

Listen to your body.

Always be mindful of what your body is saying. If you feel that the method you chose is not working for you, then stop. You can try another method. If you feel too exhausted to continue, then relax and give yourself a break. Prioritize your health always.

How to Write a Diet Plan and Follow It

Planning your meal that will coincide with your intermittent fasting goals can be quite tricky but not impossible. In fact, it can become fairly easy once you get the hang of things. To help you on your way, here are some helpful tips on how you can write your diet plan:

Keep things personal.

Before you write your diet plan, you need to do some self-reflection first. It is important that you examine your needs and views on the entire IF approach to develop the best meal plan for you. Identify the nitty gritty details of your plans first before you begin writing your diet plans such as your views regarding exercising, eating, preferred foods, and more.

Choose the right method.

Decide on which method of intermittent fasting you are most comfortable following. As a woman, you need to take extra care in your choices because the effects are far diverse than those of men when you choose the wrong approach. If you are in doubt, always ask your doctor or stay with the approaches that alter your routine the least.

Set a calorie limit.

Although intermittent fasting is not really focused on the specific number of calories per day, it is recommended that you keep your calories in check. If you are a slightly inactive woman, one trick you can do to determine the required daily calories for you is to multiply your weight (in pounds) to 10. If you are relatively active, then multiply by 12. Once you get your average calories per day, cut about at least 400 to 500 calories from that on your fasting days.

Load on nutrients.

Keep your meals as healthy as possible. Load on lean proteins, easy-to-burn carbs, essential fats, and vitamins. Do away from processed and preserved foods as much as possible and consume lean meats, beans, nuts, fruits and vegetables, and other healthy meals.

Make things simple and easy.

If you make your diet plan too complex, at the end of the day, you will end up losing interest because of how complicated the plan is. Make meals simple. You don't have to eat gourmet just to get the maximum nutritional value. You don't also have to spend long hours with preparation. Most women fail to follow diet plans because the meals take time to cook. If you cannot allot more than an hour of your time to prepare your meals, then it is best to keep your meals easy and simple to make. Just remember to never sacrifice the quality.

Plan meals beforehand.

Plan your meals beforehand. You must set your meals for tomorrow beforehand to make sure that you don't end up making wrong food choices. It is also ideal if you can prepare meals for the next day the day before. This will keep you from eating junk and can considerably save you time.

Commit.

Some women quit following their diet plans because they feel like they are not achieving anything or perhaps they can no longer sustain the lifestyle. If you commit to your goals from day one and discipline yourself to endure until the end, then you will find it easier to follow the plan.

Dealing with the Common Diet Obstacles

A lot of women who started intermittent fasting end up quitting in the middle of their progress for a lot of reasons. There's this and there's that. The reason why they fail is not that they cannot beat these obstacles, but because they are not serious enough to do so. Here are the top eight most common diet obstacles and how you can beat them:

Eating out with family or friends

When your friends or family urge you to go out and have some fun, you will most likely end up eating some fast foods and drinking. If you decline, your girl pals might think it's rude or your family might think that you're ruining the fun. It's just a matter of strong your resolve is. If you are committed to your plans, you will be able to find a way to still stick to your plan without jeopardizing the fun times spent with friends and family. You can schedule one day each week as friends or family bonding time. Just make sure to schedule another day, usually the next day, to burn those extra calories after.

Love of food

When you love eating, it is quite difficult to tell yourself to stop. But, you must. However, it does not mean that by fasting, you completely forget your love of food. You can still eat your favorite foods, but only in limited portions.

Lack of commitment

Some women quit their diet because they cannot commit. Some women only try out fasting because it's the trend. Your friend's doing it, so you do it too. You are not really putting your heart and mind into your diet which makes you susceptible to quitting. If you want to do IF, then do it because you want to and not just because you must.

Occasions and events

Going on events and occasions is also another venue where you cannot control what you eat. However, that does not mean that you let go of yourself either. You can still eat the meals served but just make sure to manage what you are eating and by how much.

Too much stress

Stress is a great precursor to a lot of diseases these days. It is also one of the main reasons why people lose motivation. Learn to manage your stress. If you are too stressed at work, you won't mind much about your meals. Sometimes you end up doing emotional binge eating which is not healthy and derails your progress. So, spend the time to relax and just relieve yourself of too much stress. A jog in the park is a great way to keep your mind off things. Reading a good book is also a good choice.

The ideal body

Most women have a pre-conceived idea of what the ideal body of women should look like. This mindset greatly affects the way women decide on how they should proceed with their diets. Remember that every person is made unique. Being sexy is just a relative term.

Remember that in today's age, being healthy is way better than just being sexy.

Limited finances

Money can also be a great factor when it comes to dieting. Someday that they cannot follow those healthy recipes because the ingredients are too expensive. It doesn't have to be that way. Money doesn't have to be an issue when it comes to dieting. In fact, going on a diet should be able to help improve your finances since you are cutting on food consumption. If you cannot buy the ingredients, then grow them yourself. Having a mini garden doesn't only help you minimize the expenses, it can also help you relax.

Lack of time

Some women who go on an intermittent fasting diet find it difficult to proceed because of lack of time.

Well, lack of time is not the problem here. It's how you manage time. If you can plan your meals right, time your fasting hours right, then you won't have to deal with problems regarding time management. Tweak your plan until you can find a suitable schedule that you can easily adapt and follow.

Conclusion

As a woman, there are a lot of diet fads out there that serve nothing but as clutter. These diet fads claim to do this, do that, only to run short. Intermittent fasting is not like those. Intermittent fasting is backed with years of studies and science to be able to claim the benefits that it offers. If you engage in intermittent fasting, you are given a chance to improve your health and your life.

Whether your aim is to lose weight, maintain healthier skin, decrease the risk of developing diseases, or something else, intermittent fasting can get you there. This book will serve as your springboard to get started on that journey. May the things that you learned in this book serve as your guide in starting your quest as a beginner at intermittent fasting.

About the Co-Author

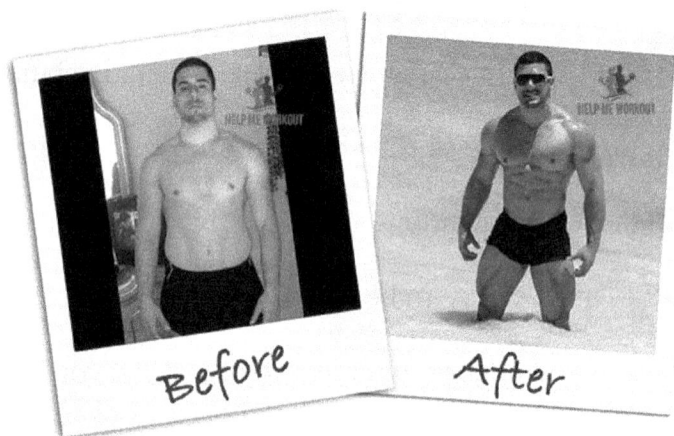

Before   After

My name is George Kaplo; I'm a certified personal trainer from Montreal, Canada. I'll start off by saying I'm not the biggest guy you will ever meet, and this has never really been my goal. In fact, I started working out to overcome my biggest insecurity when I was younger, which was my self-confidence. This was due to my height measuring only 5 foot 5 inches (168cm), it pushed me down to attempt anything I ever wanted to achieve in life. You may be going through some challenges right now, or you may simply want to get fit, and I can certainly relate.

For me personally, I was always kind of interested in the health & fitness world and wanted to gain some muscle due to the numerous bullying in my teenage years about my height and my overweight body. I figured I couldn't do anything about my height, but I sure can do something about how my body looked like. This was the beginning of my transformation journey. I had no idea where to start, but I just got started. I felt worried and afraid at times that other people would make fun of me for doing the exercises the wrong way. I always wished I had a friend that was next to me who was knowledgeable enough to help me get started and "show me the ropes."

After a lot of work, studying and countless trial and errors. Some people began to notice how I was getting more fit and how I was starting to form a keen interest in the topic. This led many friends and new faces to come to me and ask me for fitness advice. At first, it seemed odd when people asked me to help them get in shape. But what kept me going is when they started to see changes in their own body and told me it's the first time that they saw real results! From there, more people kept coming to me, and it made me realize after so much reading and studying in this field that it did help me, but it also allowed me to help others. I'm now a fully certified personal trainer and have trained numerous clients to date who have achieved amazing results.

Today, my brother Alex Kaplo (also a Certified Personal Trainer) and I own & operate this publishing venture, where we bring passionate and expert authors to write about health and fitness topics. We also run an online fitness website "HelpMeWorkout.com" and I would love to connect with by inviting you to visit the website on the following page and signing up to our e-mail newsletter (you will even get a free book).

Last but not least, if you are in the position I was once in and you want some guidance, don't hesitate and ask... I'll be there to help you out

Your friend and coach,

George Kaplo

Certified Personal Trainer

Get another book for Free

I want to thank you for purchasing this book and offer you another book (just as long and valuable as this book), "Health & Fitness Mistakes You Don't Know You're Making", completely free.

Visit the link below to signup and receive it:

www.hmwpublishing.com/gift

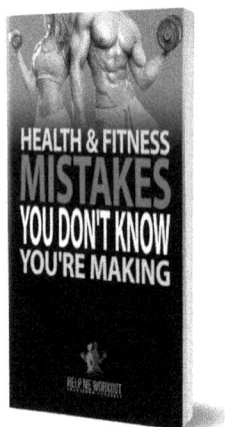

In this book, I will break down the most common health & fitness mistakes, you are probably committing right now, and I will reveal how you can easily get in the best shape of your life!

In addition to this valuable gift, you will also have an opportunity to get our new books for free, enter giveaways, and receive other valuable emails from me. Again, visit the link to sign up: www.hmwpublishing.com/gift

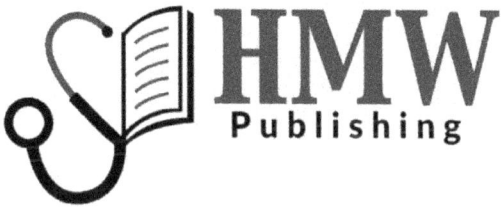

For more great books visit:

HMWPublishing.com

www.ingramcontent.com/pod-product-compliance
Lightning Source LLC
Chambersburg PA
CBHW050732030426
42336CB00012B/1520